How To Lose Weight by Speeding Up Your Metabolism

Foods that Speed Up Your Metabolism and Metabolism Boosters

CASEY STARK

ISBN-13: 978-1507537367
ISBN-10: 1507537360

CONTENTS

1. INTRODUCTION

What if there was a fat burning machine that would burn off your excess weight for you, completely free and you didn't even have to go on a diet or even eat less? Well, there is! It's inside you working away right now, burning calories and it's called your metabolism.

Your metabolism burns off over half of the fat and energy your body uses every day without you even thinking about it or probably even knowing it.

We can easily boost the built in fat burning ability of our bodies to help us burn off even more excess weight by simply eating regularly and choosing more foods that boost our metabolisms.

If you have a faster metabolism, you will use more calories even when resting. It's that simple and you know what they say about simple ideas, they're the best!

The best thing about this is that your metabolism never stops, it's literally 24/7. So if you speed it up, you will be literally burning fat in your sleep.

In this guide I will take you through everything you need to know about how exactly your metabolism works to increase your understanding and help you better grasp the science behind the system.

I will explain how your metabolism is totally unique to you as an individual, what to eat for breakfast, lunch and dinner, what to avoid and even some motivational tips.

I literally have everything covered in this one easy guide to get you clued up and on the path to easy, fast weight loss that is backed up by science and actually does work.

2. WHAT IS YOUR METABOLISM?

Metabolism is the word for the chemical transformations in the cells of inside your body. The word metabolism, when talking about digestion, refers to the transportation of substances into and between different cells.

Put simply, your food is broken down by your body and the nutrients are absorbed. Enzymes in your digestive system make these chemical transformations possible and release energy stored in the food that you have eaten.

Metabolism does not only refer to breaking down and releasing energy from your food however, it also refers to the processes that use those nutrients to repair and build our bodies.

The vast majority of the energy we use every day, we use without even knowing it. This is because much is needed to keep our bodies functioning normally and rebuild our bodies.

These two separate parts of your metabolism are called catabolism and anabolism.

To be more precise catabolism refers to be breakdown of the food that you eat. Be it carbohydrates, proteins or fats so that they can be used by the body for both energy and to build and re-build our bodies.

Anabolism refers to the part of our metabolism that does the building and repairs of our bodies. The amount of energy needed by your Anabolism is the minimum you need to consume to maintain a consistent weight.

If you consume more energy than the amount that your anabolism needs, and you're not burning off that excess with exercise, it will be stored by your body as fat.

The energy that is released from our food via our digestive systems is measured in kilojoules. The amount of kilojoules that our bodies use or burn over time is dictated by our metabolism and our metabolic rate.

So our metabolism is perhaps the single most important factor in losing and gaining weight. If we can learn to not control but at least influence our metabolism, we can use this to great advantage when trying to alter our body fat levels.

3. HOW IS YOUR METABOLISM UNIQUE

Metabolisms are unique to everyone and every living organism on the planet. Your metabolic system is what determines what substances your body will be able to use as food and what it will reject or find poisonous. This is why we can eat chocolate for example, yet it is poisonous to dogs.

Your metabolism is effected by various factors such as how old you are, your gender, the amount of physical activities you engage in and your weight. Both muscle weight and fat weight effect your metabolism.

Of course another factor that has a major effect on your metabolism is the food you eat, which of course I will be covering thoroughly in this book.

The main factors that will control your metabolism however are your hormones and your nervous system.

There are three main parts of your metabolic rate and they are individual to us all. These are important to understanding how this all works so pay close attention on this part! The three main components of metabolic rate are as follows.

BMR or basal metabolic rate. This refers to the total kilojoules of energy that your body burns when you are resting. Basal metabolic rate is basically the same thing as your anabolism. This perhaps surprisingly accounts for the majority of your energy expenditure, about 50 to 80 percent.

As with everything to do with your metabolism your BMR is personal to you. A major factor in the amount of energy your BMR uses is your lean muscle mass. So, if you have more muscle, you will burn more calories naturally. If you aren't very muscular and eat the same amount, that leaves more left over energy for your body to turn into fat.

It is important to try to increase your lean muscle mass if you are trying to lose weight in order to burn more energy and fat naturally.

To give you a rough idea, the average man's BMR is about 7000 kJ a day and an average woman's BMR is about a thousand or so less.

The second part is the energy that you use during physical activity. This should account for over 20 per cent of your energy use for an average non-strenuous day. So obviously if you work in a physical job or you're an active person in general this could be considerably higher than in other people who lead a less active lifestyle.

For those of you who exercise or have an extremely active job, energy expenditure from physical activity should at least double. The exact amount is extremely difficult to predict due to the amount of variables such as age, weight and the amount of physical exertion the particular activity takes.

As a rough guide, during an hour long fairly intense physical activity you could burn though up to 3000 kJ an hour.

The third and final part is the thermic effect of food. Obviously your food doesn't just enter your body and magically turn into energy, a percentage of the energy you have previously metabolized is required to do this. So basically, this is the energy that is used to actually eat, digest and metabolize your food.

The thermic effect of food therefore increases your BMR. After eating your BMR will rise and start to use energy more rapidly to digest your food over the next few hours.

Some foods have a greater thermic effect than others and will therefore burn energy faster, this of course has to be balanced with the energy content of the food.

All of these factors contribute to your personal metabolism are unique to each and every one of us.

Now that we have this information we can begin to take control of our own unique metabolisms and tailor its speed to suit our needs.

4. HOW SPEEDING UP YOUR METABOLISM CAN HELP YOU LOSE WEIGHT

The speed of your metabolism is known as your metabolic rate. The metabolic rate of any living organism dictates how much food it will need.

This is important because if we consume more kilojoules of energy than our basal metabolic rate allows, and if we do not burn off this excess of energy via exercise and physical activities, the energy is stored by our bodies as fat.

If you want to lose weight then obviously a higher BMR means more of the energy is being burnt off without us even needing to do anything!

The best thing about this is that diets can actually have a negative effect on weight loss programs that are based around fast metabolism weight loss programs.

In fact I think in most cases, dieting is more trouble than it's worth. Don't get me wrong though I'm not saying don't eat healthily, I'm just saying that people get it wrong a lot of the time and don't really understand them properly.

For example if you diet on its own and that's all you're trying to do to lose weight then that's usually not overly effective. This is due to the fact that your body will realize it's not getting the amount of energy it needs and will slow down your metabolism to compensate.

Then you're eating very little and/or the food you are eating probably doesn't taste very nice and your metabolism is actively working to try and save as much energy as it can which is the opposite of what you want it to do.

This is why, I won't even call it a diet, an eating plan that will boost your metabolism is by far the best option in my opinion.

5. THINGS TO AVOID

As I have already mentioned, dieting in the traditional sense of eating less food and therefore taking in less fuel and energy for your body will slow down your metabolism. So avoid dieting at all costs.

If at all possible, try not to be female. Sorry ladies but you generally have a lower BMR than men meaning that you need less energy for your bodies to run. Also remember what I said about muscle being a good fat burner? Women generally have less muscle. Handy if you're stuck on a desert island, not handy if you like eating.

Alcohol can have an effect on our metabolisms too because it effects the transportation of fats as they are being digested. This results in more fat being taken into the blood stream and therefore, more weight gain.

Due to modern lifestyles people seem to eat here and there and not very much throughout the day and then have one large meal when they get home. Some people even skip breakfast which I can't understand for the life of me!

Now in this guide I'm going to tell you to eat a lot but having one excessively large meal can actually slow down your metabolism. This is due to the effect it has on your insulin levels.

Insulin is released by your body when glucose levels in your blood stream rise. This lets the cells in your body know if they can store some of the energy for a later date in the form of fat.

Having a large meal and eating a lot in one go will increase the glucose levels in your blood, which in turn releases more inulin, which tells your body to get storing that energy away and put on the pounds.

6. BREAKFAST

Now this is important… don't skip breakfast! You need to get up and kick start your metabolism straight away. If I could tell you to eat in your sleep I would.

If you skip breakfast your metabolism will start to slow down. This is due to a little evolutionary mechanism that recognizes you haven't eaten anything and starts slowing down the processes to do with digestion.

This is for two reasons. The first is to conserve as much energy as possible because it's not sure when you will next eat, just like back when we were hunter gatherers and couldn't just go down the shop for a loaf of bread. The second is because, as there's nothing to metabolize, there no reason for your metabolism to be active.

Remember, whenever your metabolism isn't acting at maximum capacity, fewer kilojoules of energy of being burned off naturally by your body and if any of that energy isn't needed right away it will be stored as fat.

Now, I'm not talking about having a dry piece of toast and a glass of water. The reason for this is that studies have found, people who have a larger meal at breakfast put on far less weight on average than people who ate less. This is the beauty of this way of losing weight, and why it's so popular, you can practically stuff your face. Just try not to eat total rubbish.

So here's some statistics for you. People that consumed between 22-55 percent of their total daily calories in the morning put on 1.7 pounds on average after four years, I know that's putting on weight but the next stat will make you realize the significance of this. People who consumed between 0-11 percent of the daily calories they would consume all day first thing in the morning, they gained just under 3 pounds over the same time period.

Also, people involved in the same study who skipped breakfast on a regular basis increased their chances of obesity 4.5 times over! So yeah, breakfast really is the most important meal of the day!

The best foods to eat in the morning are foods that will digest slowly. Complex carbohydrates are hard for your metabolism to break down so will digest slowly which is perfect. Lean proteins are great for breakfast too and fat is fine as long as it's the healthy kind and not saturated fats.

As a general rule you want to stay away from pastries like croissants etc. A much better choice is whole grain cereal. Eggs are great too as they're a good source of protein and provide a decent dose of energy to get your metabolism fired up for the day.

Lean protein is great for your metabolism. A good source of healthy protein, and no I'm not getting paid to say this and other meat substitutes are available, is Quorn. Meat offers a good amount of protein but generally contains a decent amount of fat. Also red meat, which is generally what people eat for breakfast, is just really bad for you to be honest. So Quorn and other meat substitutes are fantastic sources of extremely healthy protein with a far lower fat content than meat and are brilliant for metabolism boosting!

Oats are a fantastic source of carbohydrates that are a classic, all-time favorite breakfast food. Oats do contain some protein too, a very small amount of fat, but mainly lots of carbohydrates to keep your metabolism working away in the background. Oats are also a great source of fiber, which leads me nicely on to my next topic where fiber plays a big part.

Now I'm not a big fan of fruit personally but both fruits and vegetables are full of fiber. Apart from being good for your digestive system in general, fiber is an excellent natural fat burner. Fiber also regulates your blood sugar, which as I mentioned earlier in the book is very important to weight loss as if your blood sugar goes up, your insulin levels rise and your body starts to store some of the glucose in your blood as fat. So fiber in general is extremely important.

If you're like me and you're not fruit lover then you can always find ways to make them taste a bit nicer by mixing it with yoghurt or chopping it up and adding it to your cereal. Or of course my personal favorite and the best way to eat fruit ever, smoothies!

As for dairy products, most diets will tell you they are a no go area because of the high fat content. However, with the metabolism boosting system, dairy can be a great addition to your diet. Low fat dairy products will give you protein which, as mentioned, will help to boost your metabolism further.

So for example, an big old omelet is a great breakfast food for your metabolism. Throw some of your favorite vegetables in there too. Bit different from most diets where they tell you to have half a bowl of muesli huh? Combine this with some porridge and you've got a great, pretty big, breakfast that will do wonders for your metabolism and get your body off to a good fat burning start to the day.

As for tea and coffee, there was a study done for that too! It's good news for my fellow caffeine drinkers. On average the metabolic rate of people who drank coffee was 16 percent higher than the other people who drank decaffeinated drinks.

The reason caffeine helps is because caffeine actually stimulates your body, your central nervous system to be precise. This may be common knowledge but caffeine's stimulating effects raise your heart rate and breathing rate. This extra work that your body is doing burns calories off without you even doing anything!

Also if at all possible, space your breakfast out. This might sound weird but if you eat too much at once your glucose levels in your blood will go up and as I have mentioned this means weight gain. So if you can have an omelet for example when you first wake up then get ready and then have the second part of your breakfast that would be beneficial.

7. LUNCH AND DINNER

So in this chapter I'm going to cover some of the metabolism boosting foods that will really help you shed the pounds!

Now lean meat is fantastic for the protein it contains. Not only does it help speed up your metabolism but it also helps you put on muscle. The more muscle you have the more energy you burn through on a daily basis even when you're just sitting about.

As I have mentioned meat substitutes, I think, are a far better way of getting the same protein levels but with a lot less fat involved. It's pretty easy to switch the chicken in your stir fry to chicken style pieces or the steak on your plate for a beef style steak.

For those of you who are set on eating meat however lets first start off let's start with salmon. You may have heard that it contains more calories than whitefish but it is low in saturated fat. Salmon is also high in protein and Omega 3.

Omega 3 is an essential fatty acid and is very healthy, so don't let the word fat put you off as not all fats are bad! Fatty acids are known as an "essential" fatty acid. Anything with essential in the name means that our bodies can't make it so we need to consume and metabolize it via our food.

Omega 3 is contained in all fish, not just salmon. Salmon is particularly high in omega 3 however as it isn't a warm water fish which tend to contain less. Omega 3 helps stop blood clots and the clogging of arteries and therefore help prevent heath attacks and strokes.

Anyway back to the point, salmon is a great source of protein and protein is very important for metabolism boosting!

Turkey is another meat that is high in protein but take the skin off because it's full of fat! Apart from boosting your metabolism protein is needed for muscle growth. This is important because, as mentioned earlier in the book, the more lean muscle you have the more calories you will burn naturally.

Now the inevitable, celery. Pretty much every diet book ever written will tell you to eat celery. Chocolate bar? Nah, on a diet… celery it is then. I have to put it in the book though because it is commonly thought of to burn off more calories during digestion than it contains. So what better food is there for a metabolism based diet? A food that not only speeds up your metabolism but that also contains so little calories that it will make you lose weight but by eating it!

Don't worry though if you're not a celery fan because there is an alternative. Melons are also fantastic food for losing weight. It has been said that the cantaloupe melon does the same job as celery in the way that it takes more energy to metabolize it than it contains.

Another food that is said to have the same effect as celery and cantaloupes is asparagus. Something that most people would find far more appealing than celery. I'm not sure if it definitely does have the same effect but it is low calorie that's for sure. It's also full of nutrients and very good for you in general and as a great source of fiber it will help keep those insulin levels in check and therefore keep the weight gain down.

So on to spicy foods! There are a variety of spices that are said to be metabolism boosters. Obviously included in this category are curries but don't go eating super fatty take away curry every day and expecting to lose weight! Other spices that are said to do wonders for your metabolism are Cinnamon, Black/Cayenne Pepper and Mustard.

These spices are great additives that add a splash of flavor to a lot of foods so whack some of them on and get eating to give your metabolism an extra boost!

Cucumber is something I'm not a fan of but it's great for our metabolism boosting strategy. Lots of good nutrients and a high fiber content with a very low calorie count. Try adding them to your sandwiches and salads and they should help you shed some weight!

Stir fry is another option that's fully on the menu for metabolism burners. The fiber in the vegetables and lean protein in the meat (which I highly recommend switching for a meat substitute such as Quorn for the super low fat protein) are great together for boosting your metabolism. You definitely want to try throwing some ginger in there too because ginger has been shown to have fantastic metabolism increasing properties

Red Beans are another great metabolism booster. Beans are a common diet food because they are widely known to increase your metabolism. Resistant starch that is found in red beans has been found to help lower your insulin levels and therefore causes your body to store less energy and put on less fat.

B vitamins that are also found in red beans is a testosterone booster, which is definitely a good thing. The reason testosterone levels are important is because a higher testosterone level means more muscle. The more muscle you have the more energy you will burn even while resting.

Another tip is that dried beans are better for you that the canned ones, they aren't as convenient as you will have to soak them before cooking and eating them but it's worth it.

They are very easy to incorporate into your diet as you can just eat them with whatever else you're having really! Having soup? Whack some beans in. Having Toast? Whack some beans on. Having beans? Have some extra beans. Easy.

As for drinks, as I already mentioned, caffeine is great for speeding up your whole body and burning calories. Green tea is also something you should consider. There was a study that found people who were given green tea and caffeine used more calories than people who were given a placebo or caffeine alone.

8. SNACKS

You ideally want to be snacking throughout the day to keep your metabolism at peak performance and stop yourself being very hungry at meal times so you don't binge eat.

Also if you do snack throughout the day you won't be as likely to get cravings for junk food or foods that you shouldn't be eating.

So here are some great snack ideas for speeding up your metabolism.

Nuts are fairly high in fat so don't go crazy on them but you can chop them and have them with yoghurt for example. Nuts help burn fat and boost your metabolism because they turn the thyroid hormone into its active form. They even take care of the toxins that build up in your fat cells and cause cellulite! The other great thing about them is that they are a fantastic source of protein. The protein will provide a thermic effect which means your body will be burning more calories to digest it.

Avocados are another great food to snack on throughout the day. They also contain fat but as it's monounsaturated fat, it actually provides 3 fat burning effects to help with weight loss. The first is that it helps call membranes work better with the fat-burning hormones that are present in your body. The second effect is that it protects the areas of your cells that produce energy from damage from free radicals. The third and main thing though is that it actually decreases the effect of hormones that tell your body to store fat.

Although not technically a snack, you can definitely eat them as a snack throughout the day. Chia seeds are fantastic for suppressing your appetite. They also burn fat naturally by the use of glucagon which is a fat burning hormone naturally created by your body.

Obviously fruit is fantastic for your health in general. Just remember fruit helps to regulate your insulin levels and stop your body packing away too much energy as fat.

Berries are a great tasting, fiber packed insulin regulator and can be made into smoothies which will help make you feel more full. They are also great for health in general so go crazy!

Grapefruit in particular possesses chemicals that promote weight loss. The vitamin C it contains is great for reducing insulin levels which will also help you lose weight. They also help reduce food cravings. Research has found that people who have a glass of grapefruit juice or a whole grapefruit before a meal burn off on average and additional 3 pounds in just 12 weeks.

Various healthy oat bars are on the market right now. I have already gone into why oats are great for your metabolism but they release energy slowly so make a great snack.

As mentioned before, as well as snacking you should be keeping topped up on your caffeine. If you drink coffee or other caffeinated drinks you will naturally produce more adrenaline. Adrenaline actually tells your busy to get busy burning fat so it's pretty important!

9. HANDY TIPS

A great tip that you can incorporate easily into your everyday life is to chill your water or add ice. Water is great in general and a study found that volunteers who drank more water had higher metabolic rates than others. Drinking your water cold causes your body to heat it up, this takes energy to do and that energy would otherwise be left floating around your body and if not burned off it would turn to fat so can only help your efforts!

Obviously the amount of calories you will burn from drinking cold water won't be much but research has shown that drinking 5 glasses of ice cold water a day can lose 5 pounds over the course of a year. So if you make a habit of it then over time it will help and as it's such an easy thing to do I would definitely recommend it.

Remember to try and eat foods that contain vitamin B as it help you metabolize your food. When you don't have enough vitamin B your metabolism will slow down. Foods that will help with this are beans, spinach, broccoli, eggs and melon.

Magnesium is very important to keep in mind. It not only

helps your metabolism run at optimum performance. It's also one of the main minerals that experts say we don't get enough of. To get a good magnesium boost, green vegetables are they key such as spinach. Spinach is easy to incorporate into your diet, it can go in soups for example and even if you don't like it you will hardly know it's there!

If you're going to be working out then short intense workouts can be great to help speed up your metabolism. An intense workout of say 20-30 minutes has been shown to help burn fat extremely effectively and actually be better at helping shed the pounds than spending hours doing a slow measured workout routine.

There are many workout programs out at the moment that you may have seen advertised on TV. They boast short intense workouts that you can fit into your everyday routine even if you're busy. The best thing about these workout DVD's is that they can help you stay motivated to stay on top of your fitness rather than just trying to motivate yourself.

10. WHAT NOT TO EAT

Carbohydrates are a huge part of most people's diets. A simple rule to follow however is to try to stick to carbohydrates that aren't white. White bread, pasta and rice are refined and have had the complex carbohydrates removed meaning your body doesn't have to use as much energy to metabolize them. Aside from this, they contain far less of the good nutrients as a lot of them have been removed. Try switching to brown bread and pasta for a double hit health/metabolism boost.

Pesticides have been said to have a detrimental effect on the speed of our metabolisms. Try to eat organic fruit and vegetables wherever possible.

The foods that tend to contain the most pesticides are apples, spinach, lettuce, cucumber, potatoes, green beans, celery, strawberries, peaches and grapes.

The ones that tend to contain the lower level of pesticides however are onion, mangoes, kiwi, grapefruit, pineapple, watermelon, mushrooms, avocado, sweetcorn, cabbage and asparagus.

Sugary foods will cause an increase in the glucose levels in your blood. As mentioned this causes an insulin increase and causes you to store the glucose as fat. Fruit is a much better option for satisfying a sugar craving.

Obviously fatty foods are generally something you will want to avoid when losing weight. Most foods that slow your metabolism do so because they are easily digested and require less energy to metabolize. When you eat fat your metabolism simply doesn't know what to do with it all and slows down to let your body start working on storing the fat to use in the future when if needs it.

So fat not only slows your metabolism but it also causes you to put on weight. The best thing to do to avoid fat easily is to not fry your food in oil and only eat foods with a high fat content like cheese in moderation.

11. WORKING OUT A DIET PLAN

The beauty of this way of eating, is that you don't necessarily need a diet plan. You can just keep in mind the information that you have learnt in this book and eat the food that you now know will speed up your metabolism.

If you want faster results and you would like to get a bit more in depth however, you can work out the calories that you should be eating.

The first step to working out a diet plan to lose weight based on your metabolism is by working out roughly what your basal metabolic rate or BMR is.

As mentioned earlier in the book, this is the name for the standard rate of your metabolism while you are resting.

To work out your BMR there is a few calculations you need to do so get a pen and paper!

For women take your weight in pounds and multiply it by 4.35. Then add this to your total height in inches multiplied by 4.7. Then add 655 and finally minus your age multiplied by 4.7.

So it would look like this:

655 + (4.35 x weight) + (4.7 x height) - (4.7 x age)

For men take your weight in pounds and multiply it by 6.23. Then add this to your total height in inches multiplied by 412.7. Then add 66 and finally minus your age multiplied by 6.8.

Which would look like this:

BMR = 66 + (6.23 x weight) + (12.7 x height) - (6.8 x age)

The number that you get will be a decent guideline to what your BMR is. This will tell you how many calories you need be consuming on a daily basis.

So if you're doing nothing to alter your metabolism as you would with a traditional style diet and you're not exercising you have to lower your calorie intake so it's below the number you just calculated.

With a metabolism boosting diet, you don't have to eat less calories unless you want to speed up your weight loss further, you simply have to eat the right foods.

If you exercise then obviously the calorie total you can consume will be different. For example if you exercise heavily on a daily basis you should double the number you got.

So to sum up, take the number you got from the calculation and try to stick somewhere around that number as far as your calorie intake goes and as long as you're eating metabolism boosting foods, you will be losing weight without having to go on a diet. Add in some exercise and you will be losing weight even faster!

12. DIETARY SUPPLEMENTS AND PILLS

We are living in a world that has created a thirst for media that is exposing us to more trends is society than ever before.

One trend that seems to stick decade after decade in the modern world is to look slim and fit. The curvy look is only considered appealing to the media when it comes with a very slim waistline. This is something that has made a lot of men and women obsessive about their weight and start to look for the best supplements and pills they can find in order to get a body that looks exactly like the one on the cover of the magazines.

There are many ways to lose weight and some of them involve more sacrifices than others. Some people choose to get surgery to remove fat and to tone their bodies, but that is a temporary solution if you don't have a good diet to go with it. Other buy expensive treatments and even get hypnotherapy in order to stop eating junk food and lose weight, but this is also not going to be so useful if you don't work out and do all kinds of fat burning exercises that will tone your body as you lose weight.

We have seen an even newer method for weight loss that has gained popularity in the last decade and that is the use of metabolism increasing supplements and that are supposed to turn your body into a fat burning machine by just taking them alone. In some cases they even claim that you won't even need to go on a diet because the pills will keep the fat from being absorbed by your body and you will not gain weight even if you at greasy food.

The truth is that this pills might not be harmful for your body in any way that should raise any alarms, but if someone abuses their use they could suffer from blood pressure problems, dehydration, mood swings and insomnia. Some people report digestive problems too, but the biggest issue with these pill is that they don't really work as they should.

When you lose fat while you take diet pills, you will usually be given the advice of going on a healthy diet and also doing plenty of exercise. This is the method that most of those fat burning pills use because they know you will lose some fat by changing your diet and exercising even if you don't take their pill. This is the perfect way to cover up the lack of results that a pill can provide on its own.

In conclusion you need to understand that there is no such thing as a perfect fat burning pill that is going to get rid of all of your body fat. You need to go on a diet and you need to learn to eat foods that can help you burn fat and increase your metabolism naturally by splitting your servings into smaller but more frequent meals and eating metabolism boosting foods.

There is no way to lose weight because of a pill alone. The pills can help suppress your appetite, but they will not act as fat burners. If those pills actually worked as they are advertised to work, most gyms would be out of business within months!

If you do decide to take a weight loss pills I strongly recommend that you always check with your doctor before you decide to take any kind of pill or go on a diet. Your health should always be your priority and even when you are trying to lose weight, you need to be careful on the methods you use to accomplish this goal.

13. THE MYTHS OF METABOLISM DIETS

As with most dieting tips these days, the internet is full of people with opinions. Some of these opinions are based on fact and given by people who are knowledgeable on the subject they are talking about. Some other, well, they're not.

So don't believe everything you hear and read. A lot of dietary myths are old wives tales and are extremely outdated.

Sometimes it seems like as soon as people hear something they find interesting they believe it without really questioning it and then tell other people! So I thought I would add this chapter in to help you figure out the fact from the fiction.

A lot of people seem to think that people who are larger or "fatter" naturally have a slower metabolism. This isn't true.

Some thin people do seem to be able to eat whatever they want and never put on weight, that is true. This is very commonly attributed to a fast metabolism.

In fact, skinnier people almost always tend to have a slow metabolism than larger folks. This is because there is less body mass to maintain and so there is less work for the metabolism to do to power the smaller body.

This doesn't mean that if you're larger your metabolism will be going crazy burning off extra calories though, as I mentioned earlier in the book, it's mainly muscle mass that burns off calories even when you're resting.

This is a generalization we can make, people with more muscle do have higher metabolic rates than normal.

So basically, body mass does factor in to your metabolic rate but it's mainly the ratio of muscle to body size that has the greatest impact.

Another common myth you may have heard is that eating late at night or late in the evening causes you to gain weight.

There are so many factors that come into play when considering this statement that it's impossible to say eating after say 9pm will cause you to put on weight. In fact eating a meal late in the evening is pretty much exactly the same as eating at any other time throughout the day.

You're still putting the same amount of energy into your body no matter what time you eat. It's the same as any other kind of energy transference. If you change your phone late at night it's still going to have the same amount of battery as if you charge it any other time of day.

Another myth is that metabolism diets are all about food consumption. Food is obviously a great way of effecting your metabolism and makes a big difference. Something a lot of people forget however is that your metabolism is influenced by a lot of other factors.

Obviously exercise has a big impact on your metabolism and so does sleep. Research has found that people who sleep less tend to have less of an ability to control their blood sugar levels and as a consequence may find themselves feeling hungry faster than other people.

Don't forget to drink cold water and caffeine too!

14. HOW TO STICK TO YOUR DIET PLAN AND STAY MOTIVATED

In all types of diet, you may be tempted to go off the rails and indulge in something that will undo some of the hard work you have put in, even if the diet is as easy as this one! So here are a few handy tips to keep yourself motivated.

Setting yourself realistic goals is a great way to give yourself something to aim for that is a bit more short term. Short term goals will keep you on track every step of the way rather than having to aim at something that is months or years away.

There's nothing wrong with having a long term goal too but by breaking it down into monthly goals you are more likely to not slip up as you will be thinking that you don't have long left until your goal date so you will be more likely to be good!

Remember to keep your goals realistic. There's no point in setting a bunch of goals that are unachievable and not hitting them because that will do nothing for your confidence, in fact it will probably do the opposite.

You're more likely to get sick of a diet and give up in a

spectacular fashion by indulging in something you really shouldn't if you jump straight in. You don't have to suddenly jump into a diet and change everything you eat to fit it. Getting into things gradually is fine too and will help you stick to it.

If you keep going off the rails then a great way to kick your butt into shape is to write down every single thing you eat and the rough amount of calories in it. Total up your calories at the end of each day and read back over it once a week. That way, by looking back you will notice how much extra calories the little slip ups are costing you.

Hindsight is a wonderful thing and the next time you're tempted, you will remember looking back over the last few slip ups and this should help your self-control a great deal.

This isn't to say you can't eat chocolate and deserts with a metabolism based diet. Just have them in moderation. If you frustrate yourself by cutting out all of the foods you enjoy most you will be far more likely to give in.

If you do eat unhelpful foods just try to have smaller portions and eat them less often. Also, don't just wolf them down, take your time with them and really enjoy them as they should been seen as a real treat.

Remember to keep in mind why you are doing what you're doing. It helps to keep a vision in your head of your ultimate goal.

Try to remember too that your family members, co-workers and friends will be sure to notice your weight loss. Thinking about this is a great way to stay motivated and remember getting that first compliment of, "Have you lost weight?" is going to be a great feeling!

The flip side of this is to tell people about your diet and not just wait for them to notice. Or you can mix it up and maybe tell just a couple of friends about it. By telling people about your diet plans you will be talking about it as they ask about your progress and cause you to be more motivated to show them that you really can do it.

Take this one step further and if you can, get a weight loss buddy! Having someone to share the process with is a great way to stay motivated. It's not only someone to talk to about your meals and your progress, but also a bit of health competition does wonders!

You should also weigh yourself every single day, even the slightest weight difference can really help motivate you.

15. FINAL THOUGHTS

I really hope this book helps you hit your weight loss goals. I'm pretty sure I packed all the best information that I could without banging on too much about stuff you don't need to know! I think my thing is going to be short books that are packed with valuable information and I think I have achieved that with this book… maybe?

I think that I will write some more books to do with metabolism and weight loss if this one is well received so keep your eyes peeled!

If you did enjoy the books and you got it on Amazon or Kindle then please consider leaving a 5 star review as they really do help me out a lot! I'm just starting out with the whole book writing thing so the only reason people would buy anything I have written is if the reviews on the book are good, so it really will help a lot!

Thanks for reading and I will hopefully speak to you all in the next book!

Printed in Great Britain
by Amazon